From Birth to Rebirth

A Teenage Pregnancy

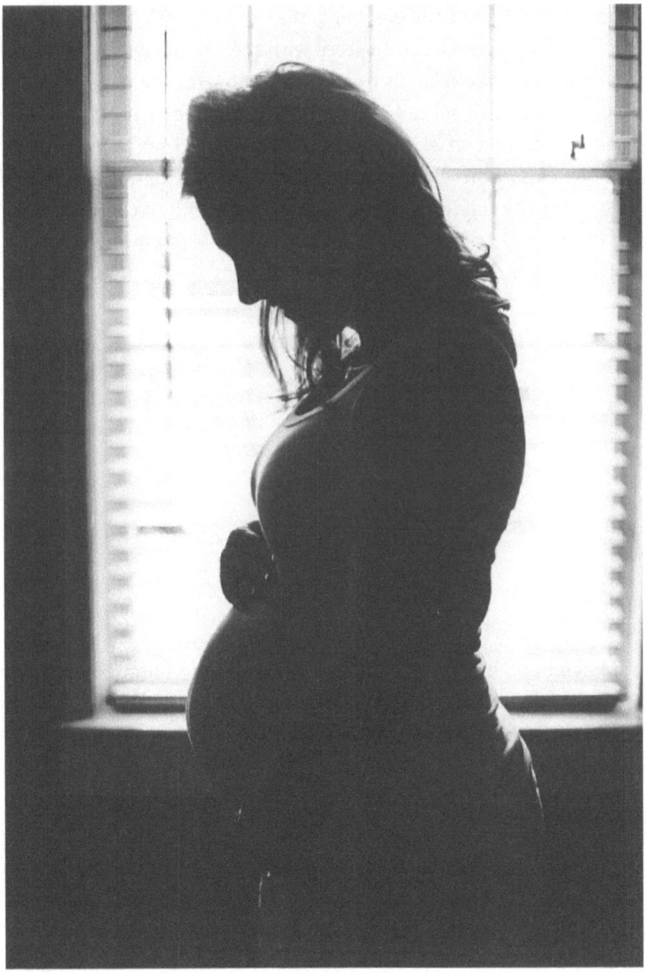

Mr. Warren,

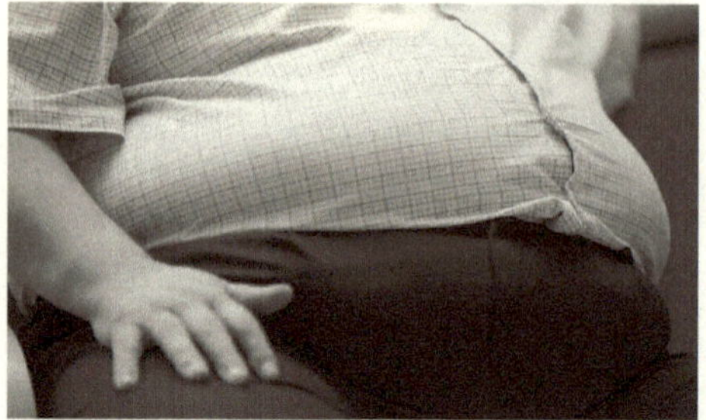

    A large man about 5'10" inches tall weighing in at an easy 400 pounds. The sweat soaked through his T-shirt as he sat on the small round stool with the metal legs he kept at the front of the classroom. The stool disappeared beneath his mass. That stool was made very well, what excellent craftsmanship. Parenting class in high school and this profusely obese man is our teacher. What an o choice. Cruel, I know but kids can be cruel and I was no exception. I sat at my desk which was located towards the back left of the classroom. 25 desks all lined up horizontally. Each desk filled with studer watching the clock waiting for the buzzer to go off signaling the end of class. Mr. Warren was listing t signs and symptoms of pregnancy on the large black board that was mounted on the wall at the fron the classroom. As he listed one by one, I followed along reading each one.

1. Fatigue

2. Bloating

3. Cramping and Pelvic Twinges

4. Missed period

5. Sore Breasts

6. Headache

It dawned on me that I have been experiencing some of those very symptoms. My heart began beati loudly, like a drum going off in my chest. It was so loud I was positive those around me could hear it. glanced around, I noticed No one was looking in my direction. I let out the breath I had not realized I holding, relieved no one noticed.

It should not have been a surprise that no one noticed me. I existed in a fog. Unnoticed, unseen...

I existed in the fog with a few stragglers that I found along the way during the first six months of high school. There were four of us including me. my palms started to sweat as I began to dread what coul possibly be something or rather someone that could change my life forever.

I always wanted to be a mom someday. but my thoughts of one day being a mom were futuristic. I w only 17 years old. I had not graduated high school or even decided what my plans for my future woul

I knew that I maybe wanted to work with young children as an Early Childhood Educator but that
s just a possibility, I have not set that as my official goal. If I was pregnant, how was I going to take
e of a tiny human. One that would rely on me for absolutely everything.

as filled with dread, as my mind raced through all the what if's I forced myself to focus. I needed to
:ide what my next step should be. But all I could think about was that I needed to tell my friends what
s going on. Like telling them made it more real. Maybe they could help me calm down and see my
4ation more clearly, perhaps i was over reacting.

rned in my desk sliding my right hand into the pocket of my favorite blue sweater I hung on the back
my chair before I sat down. I could feel my fingers wrap around what I was looking for. My life line,
' cell phone. I slowly slid it out of my pocket around the back of my chair and lowered it below the top
my desk in hopes it was out of view from the teacher. I opened my Bell Chocolate Flip phone and sent
ee texts. "Meet me in the front lobby of the school at break, it is very urgent".

er the messages were sent, I turned off my cell phone and slid it back into my sweater pocket hoping
. Warren had not noticed. There was a rule on cell phones in class. There were many rules in this
ss but the rule on cell phones in class was one of his main rules. Mr. Warren felt that cell phone use in
ss meant that we were not paying attention. his main job was to teach us and if we were not paying
ention then it made it

ficult for him to do his job. If caught with our cell phones Mr. Warren would take our phone placing
:m in a

ked drawer in his desk until the end of the school day. Not the end of his class but the end of the
1ool day. For

iny teens their cell phone as their life line. Without it they are lost.

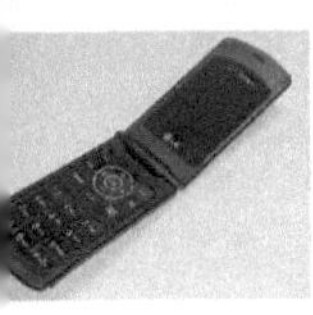

I have been at this school for three years. I have a small group of friends and never felt I need
anymore. I did not mind being alone but it is nice to have several good friends. I had gotten used to
being alone. I never realized I needed anyone other than myself until I met my three very best friends
Now I don't know how I would have gotten through high school without them. They made each day a
day to look forward to.

For years I existed in the fog alone and content. Since I started high school, I am no longer alone. I still
shuffle around lost in the fog but now I am not alone. My friends are lost in the fog with me. Before we
all had met, they too were lost alone and unnoticed just like me. They were not popular, hardly spoke
to and often ignored. Like they were lost in a fog so thick they could not be seen. We call ourselves the
fog friends. Each of us brings something unique to the group. We help lift each other up when we are
down. We help each other through problems at home and even to study for a coming test we are sure
we will fail. I needed them now more than ever.

With fifteen minutes of class left I concentrated on the clock located to the left of the door of the
classroom. The second hand ticking loudly as it went by in slow motion. The minute hand snapped like
bolts of lightning striking during a thunderstorm with each movement. Time Goes by fast when you ar
having a good time and never want it to end, but when you are anxiously waiting for time to past it
moves at a snail pace. Of course, that is an illusion, because time moves no differently either way. But
the illusion that it works to taunt us is very real.

I wonder who made the clock. How was it decided that those hands stood for seconds and
minutes. Time runs the world. The creator of the clock to tell time must have made a fortune. It is fun
the things you think about when you let your mind drift. Especially when you are trying to avoid the
reality of your own situation.

Startled, the buzzer brought me out of my trance. Finally, the end of class. Gathering my books in a fut
attempt to hurry so I did not get stuck in the usual traffic jam of students all trying to get out of the
classroom, each in a hurry for reasons all their own. The issue with being in a hurry in a classroom of
twenty-five students is that unless you are a marathon runner you will get stuck in the crowd of
students. There we were stuck squeezed together like a herd of penned up cattle grunting and groaning
each of us fighting to accomplish our goal, Freedom!

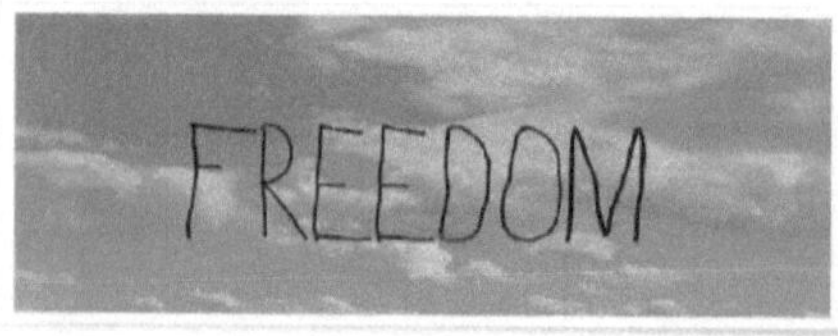

The opening of the classroom door was not very big. Maybe six feet high and four feet wide. I
not need a lot of space, just enough to squeeze through. Each day was the same no system in place
prevent the traffic jam after class when the buzzer went off. I am starting to think Mr. Warren
retly found it entertaining that we still did the same thing every day resulting in the same problem.
own little form of entertainment. While standing there trapped, my mind did what it has been doing
ce my epiphany in the beginning of class, it wandered.

This time I wondered about different scenarios like, how our very round teacher Mr. Warren
de it through the classroom door. I have never seen him enter or leave the classroom. He was just
de waiting when we arrived and left long after we did. Perhaps he turned sideways. That is the only
y it seemed possible. That had to be it. He must turn sideways to get through the door. I snapped
k into reality when I felt myself falling. Grabbing the door jamb, I steadied myself.

nding at only 4' 10" tall and weighing 130 pounds, I was able to squeeze out of tiny openings. I used
door jamb I was holding to steady myself to guide me through a small opening in front of me. Finally,
ade it through the door and into the hallway. Not only was I height impaired I was cursed with frizzy
wn hair and not just some of the time it was frizzy all the time. Our small town was humid,
rounded by three great lakes. It was a damp heat that wreaked havoc on my hair. I had thin eye
ws but they joined forming a unibrow resulting from stitches I got due to an accident when I was
ut ten years old at home.

ten used my razor to tidy it up. It was not the most ideal way to deal with it but when it but came to
metic things I did not have a lot in the way of supplies on hand or guidance on how to deal with
ngs like that. My mom was oblivious. She only saw a little girl, never noticing I was maturing and
anging. Thank God for my childhood best friend. Her name was Amy. We went our separate ways
ce we hit high school. Amy's family moved away. We kept in touch at first but not for long. I still think
her and wonder how she is doing sometimes. Amy was one year older than I was. Her mom was great
sy to talk to. She helped guide me through puberty. My mom in her defense never dealt with things
that before. So, it was all new to her. She did do better with my sister Jean.

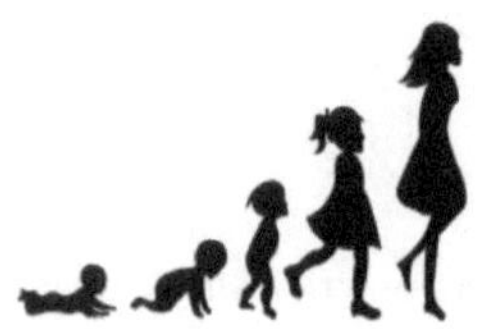

Thank Goodness. Mind you, Jean did not develop until she was fifteen years old. She was lucky in some ways and not in others. Jean and I were total opposites. I was a girlie girl and Jean was a tom boy. I was boy chasing, makeup wearing, pink curtains on the window kind of girl. Jean had sports posters on her wall and volley ball shoes tucked under the edge of her bed. We shared a room but were total opposites. We did not get along so I did my thing and Jean did Her's. Maybe one day we will find common ground and get along. We also had an older brother but he was in a category all his own.

I thought of my childhood as I walked down that hallway, lost in thought, I made my way to the front lobby of the school. At seventeen I felt I knew all there was to know and I was old enough to make decisions for myself. Mom often called me naive. Today I did question some of my latest decisions. I could see each of my friends had gotten my text and were now gathered in the front lobby waiting for me.

Standing their student filed past them as if it was empty. Lost in the fog, as if they were not existent. But at least we were not alone. We had each other. They were a great group of girls. I collected each of them within the first six months of school.

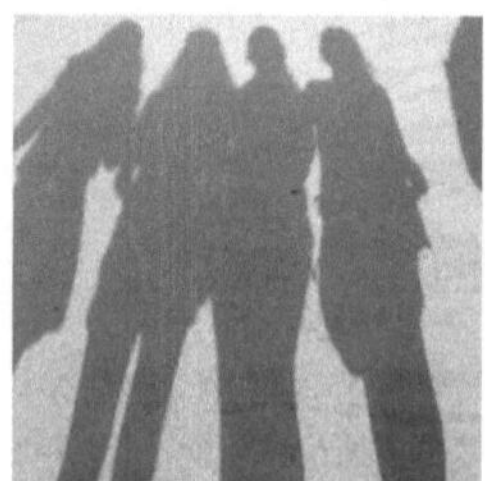

On the first day of high school my morning class was Geography. Our assignment was to take a
 of Canada and fill in all the provinces. Not my strong suit. I sat there with a blank map on my desk
ing around the classroom. Then i noticed a girl in the front of the classroom. I remember at the
nning of class the teacher had spoken to her and requested she take that seat. I also remember she
not enter class until after the announcements and morning prayer played over the school's PA
em. Juanita had dark hair and was pale. She was hard at work at her desk. I made my way with my
very blank map in hand over to her desk. Once there I leaned over the edge of her desk, said hi my
e is Lynne and began to copy her map. That was the first day of many copied assignments in that
s and the day we became friends.

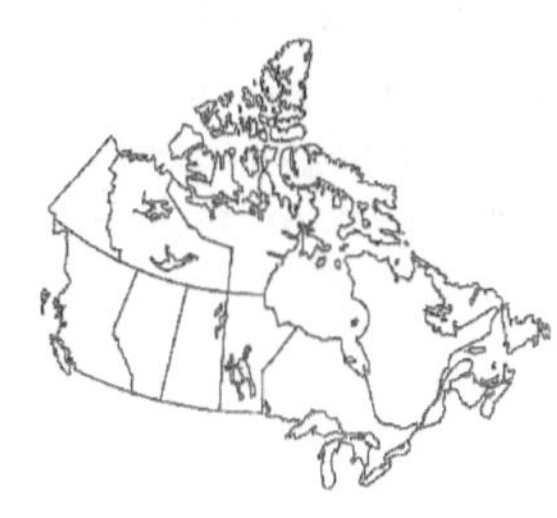

covered Juanitta's family practiced Jehovah witness as their faith. As a result, they did not watch the
s celebrate birthdays and their children did not take part in the morning announcements or the
i's prayer at school. To accommodate the school would let her stand in the hall during that part of
day. It made no sense to me as the announcements and Lord's prayer could still be heard in the
way. But to each their own.

w up going to church every Sunday. My parents took part in weekly bible studies and mom
nteered at the church soup kitchen. mom felt feeding the hungry was God's will. I was aware of
y other religions and some of their practices as Dad often spoke about various religions, he found
fascinating. Especially how some cultures were governed by their faith. There were so many
erent ones but they all did have something in common. They all believed there was good and evil
pting us. They taught right from wrong and tried to steer people down the path of good.

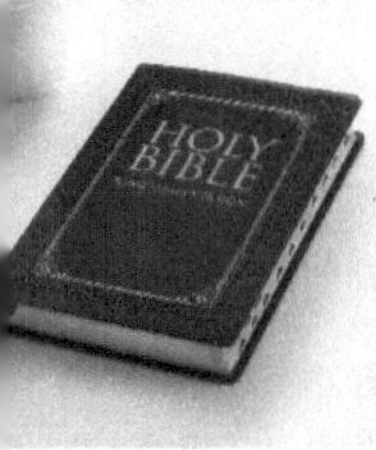

I often wondered if Juanitta and I would be friends had she not let me copy her map that morning in Geography class. I do know I would have never passed Geography class on my own. First one then one became two, Fog friends. Juanitta and I often walked the halls together on breaks between classes. Our high school was small, shaped like a square with the odd branched out hallways that dead ended and went nowhere. In the center of a gym and small outdoor smoking area.

One day on one of our many laps around the school we passed a short thin blonde that was walking close to the wall of the hallway with her head down so her hair draped over her face hiding it from view. She appeared to be making an attempt to disappear, be unnoticed. Several days went by and each day there she was. We usually ignored her and kept walking but for some reason I felt this urge to give her a little nudge with my hip as we passed. I am not sure what I was hoping to accomplish but I could not help myself. After I nudged her, she would stumble into the wall catching herself with her hands. I obviously caught her off guard. She mumbled an apology as we walked away.

I mentioned to Juanitta I found her reaction odd she did not get mad or tell me off and with some creative words. So, the next time we passed her I nudged her again. Yet a second time she stumbled, out her hands and caught herself on the nearby wall. She mumbled another apology without looking. Instead of walking away I stopped and asked her why she is apologizing that it was my fault, she should be mad and telling me off?

Again, she apologized. I decided she needed us, hooking my arm in hers I introduced Juanitta and myself. I told her we would toughen her up, so she no longer apologized for things that were not her fault. Her name was Ericka, from one to three fog friends. We were invisible to everyone else, lost in fog unseen but not alone.

The third member of our group of girls would join about six months into that first year of school. Her name was Jackie. Juanitta, Ericka and I sat at the same table every day for lunch in the school's cafeteria. That is where we met Jackie. She was seated at the other end of what we had deemed to be our table, she was being scolded like a child by what I assumed was her boyfriend. He was making a scene and she seemed embarrassed and was looking down at her lap nodding her head quietly. for some reason seeing her there like that really bothered me. Without saying a word to the others, I stood and made my way the empty chair beside her.

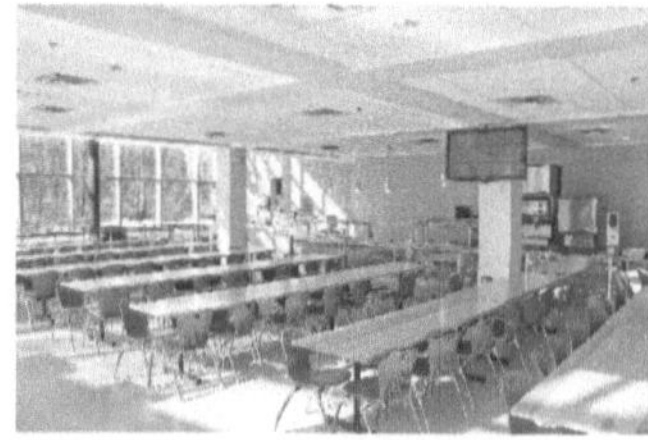

  Taking the seat, I leaned over introduced myself and informed her that she did not deserve to be treated the way the loser across the table from her was treating her. When she was ready to ditch him she could come join us. Pretending not to notice his very red face and obvious temper. I made my way back to where my friends were sitting just staring at me wide eyed with their mouths hanging open.

About a week passed before we saw Jackie again. She approached our table in the cafeteria with her head held high. She had ditched the loser and wanted to take me up on my offer to join us. From one

r. Invisible, unseen but none of us were alone in the fog. The three girls waited for me wide eyed. sure of what was so urgent that required them to meet me in the front lobby of our school. As I roached i felt a little better. It was nice to know I would not be alone no matter what. In a whisper n though no one paid attention to us I still wanted to keep it a secret I told them that i think I may be gnant. I went on to explain parenting class the list on the chalk board and how I had some of those y symptoms. Ericka was the first to speak. Her words mature and level headed. Ericka suggested I go ur local Health Unit to get a pregnancy test. She informed me that the Health Unit offers free gnancy testing, that there was no need to panic until I had a real reason to. I nodded feeling a little ter, but still felt as if I carried the weight of the world on my shoulders.

er the next few days, we would meet at classroom breaks to try and figure out the best time to go to Health Unit without missing class. If I missed the school would call my parents and all hell would ak loose. We figured out the health unit was twenty minutes each way on foot. Lunch hour was sixty utes. But I would need to take a test and it was determined there was not enough time to walk their t and make it back before lunch hour was over. Not unless I had a ride even just one way would make ifference.

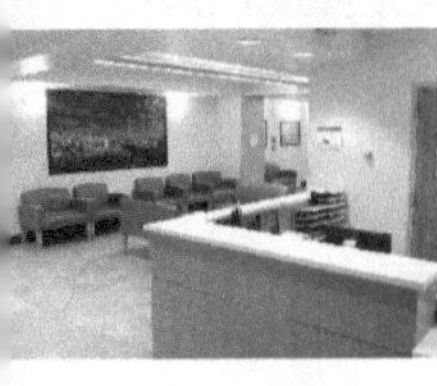

ad a boyfriend that helped me get into this mess. His name was Corey. He was tall thin with dark skin k hair and dark eyes. He was older, no longer in school and held a part time job at our local mall. He rked at the pet store doing inventory. He was kind of nerdy even considered a bad boy. But not for reasons you would think. He came from a rough family that was known to be trouble. He was not that but his reputation is the reason I dated him. He was not the kind of guy I would pick to be a dad any of my future children. Mostly because of his family. I guess I should have thought about that fore I had sex with him. I had decided if I was pregnant, I was not going to tell him. That I wanted a tter life for my baby. that my possible baby should not have to pay for mistakes. I would tell him I eated and the baby was not his. But first I needed to see I was pregnant. I arranged to meet Corey er school to see if I could borrow 20$ for cab fare. I told him it was for a doctor's appointment my m could not take me to. I was hoping to borrow the money for a cab. With no questions asked Corey nded me 20 dollars. I just hoped it was enough. After thanking him I walked home that night feeling a le bit better. things were falling into place. I just hoped the test was negative and there would be thing to tell, nothing to tell.

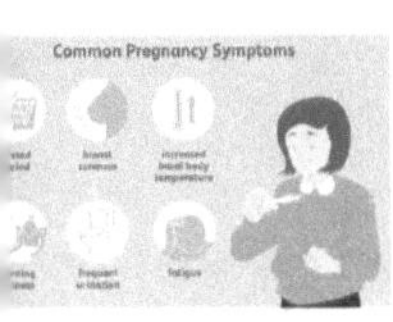

My mom would not know there was even a problem. I barely slept that night; my mind would not allow me to rest. I went through every worst-case scenario in my head. The next day at lunch I ca a cab. My friends waited outside with me for the cab to arrive. As the cab pulled up Ericka hugged me offering to come. Smiling, I told her no. If I was late for whatever reason coming back, I did not want to get into trouble. Ericka's family was strict. Her only social life was at school. She was never allowed go out or to anyone's house to visit. As the cab pulled up i took a deep breath and got in. I really hope had enough money to make it to my destination. As the cab pulled away i looked around the cab. It w old and dingy. There was a meter mounted on the dash to keep track of cost. The cab was dirty with bits of what I hoped were food crumbs on the floor boards. There were fast food wrappers on the fro passenger seat   indicating this was obviously a personal vehicle. The driver was older, slightly overweight with salt and pepper dark hair and kept looking at me through his rear-view mirror. It was unnerving.

As the cab pulled up Infront of the health Unit I noticed the meter read twelve dollars. Relieved I had enough money I handed the driver the twenty-dollar bill. I was given change, then I jumped out thank him. I felt dirty like the grime in the cab stuck to me. I went to open the door of the Health Unit but it would not budge. I noticed a paper taped to the inside of a window beside the door. It was the hours operation. Crap I never thought about the hours, if it would be open. That is one of the things I never considered when planning to come. Thank God the Health Unit was open and just closed for lunch. Ho was I going to hide this now. I would never make it back to school before lunch hour was over. Accept what I could not control I stood there looking at the building. I felt like I could not catch a break.

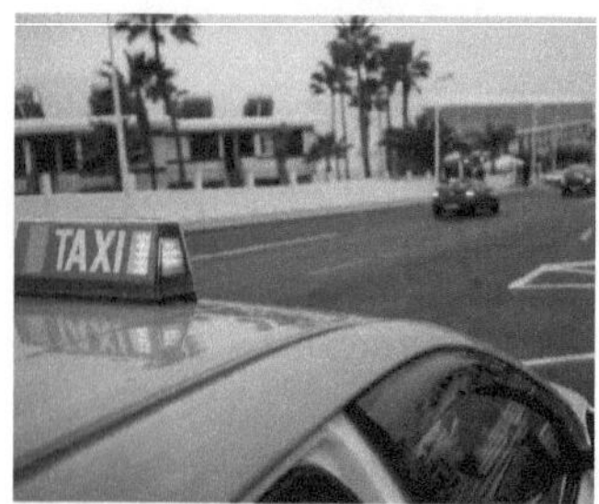

As I stood there looking around, I noticed there was a variety store just down the street. I still had a little money left from the twenty I borrowed from Corey. I also brought my school bag containin my lunch my mom packed me. Ugh... my mom. Just thinking of her made me feel sick to my stomach

essed out. freaking out now was not going to change my situation. I brushed the thought of my mom
de and walked to the variety store. I picked up some orange juice and a bag of chips.

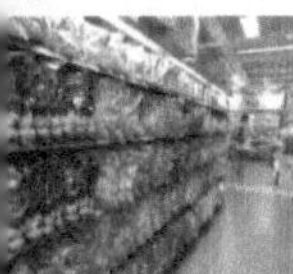

      Returning to the Health Unit, I sat by the door and ate my lunch waiting for them to open. There
s no point in turning back now. As I sat there, I thought about many random things one being about
 health Nurses that came to our school. They seemed nice enough. They came to speak about
ually transmitted disease, using protection and even brought free condoms. They discussed
gnancy and how common teen pregnancy was. They brought pamphlets with the hours of operation
ed on them and their location. I never paid much attention; I am grateful Ericka did. I never realized
y offer free pregnancy testing. I had no money to buy a test or had any idea about how much they
t. Sitting there lost in thought I never noticed the curvy grey-haired lady that was standing beside me
ng to get my attention. When she tapped my shoulder, I nearly jumped off the side walk where I was
ted. Apologizing, she asked if I needed help. I just stood there with my mouth gaping open wide
d unable to speak. I simply nodded yes. She invited me in, offered me a bottle of water and directed
 to have a seat in the waiting room. She walked to a nearby desk grabbed a clip board with papers
ped to the top and pen. Returning, she handed them to me instructing me to fill out the papers to
 best of my ability. Afterwards Leave it at the front counter and have a seat.

ere were two sheets on the clipboard, a questionnaire. One of the questions that stood out

s, when was your last period?

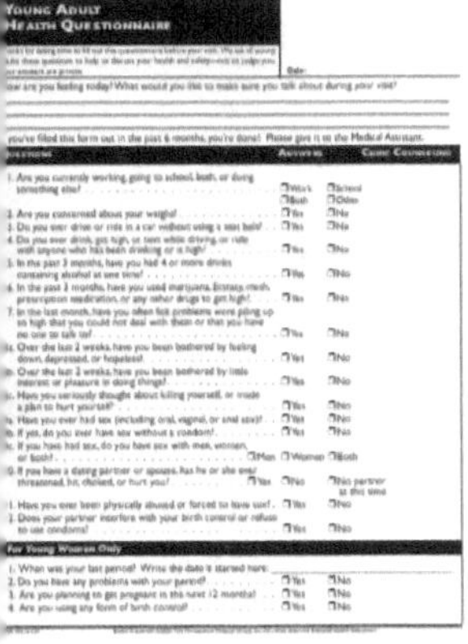

tood out like it was written there just for me. Completing the questionnaire, I placed it on the
unter then took my seat trying to wait patiently.

I waited for about fifteen minutes. Then I heard my name I listed on the questionnaire called out. I grabbed my school bag and followed the grey-haired lady to a set of double doors. Inside there was a long hallway painted mint green. On each side of the hall there were several doors. Each was closed accept one. I followed the grey-haired woman inside the only opened door. She placed the clip board the desk located in the room directing me to have a seat. Without saying another word, she walked c The room was small. Also painted mint green. There must have been a sale on that color. It had a des with a worn-out brown chair tucked in behind it. Just above the chair was a blood pressure cuff hang on the wall. There was only one place to sit. It was an old vintage-looking chair. I am not sure how lor was waiting in that small room as there was no clock to advise you of the time.

A knock at the door caught my attention. The gray-haired lady was standing in the doorway holding a box. She handed the box to me explaining it was a pregnancy test. I sat there looking at her with a bla expression on my face. She must have realized i had no idea what to do because after several minute exchanging silent looks at each other she began to explain the steps I needed to do. Afterwards she directed me to the closest bathroom down the hall. she asked that I leave the test after I had taken it the small shelf just below the bathroom mirror then return to this room and wait.

I finished with my task, returning to the room I picked up my back pack I had placed on the floor besi the door before I exited to take the test. I sat in the lone vintage chair and brought my back pack to m chest hugging it as if it somehow would protect me from my reality. I had not been waiting long wher the grey-haired lady returned.

Entering the room, she took a seat on the edge of the desk top directly across from me. In he hands were several pamphlets. She leaned towards me, placed her hand on my shoulder and told me very clearly that my pregnancy test was positive. Jumping up out of the chair in shock I shouted it had be wrong. I demanded to be retested. The lady repeated very clearly that my pregnancy test was positive. I sat back down feeling defeated. Sick to my stomach I nodded, accepting the information to true. Tears began to form as I sat there. The grey-haired lady handed me several pamphlets she was holding. She began to explain what my options were.

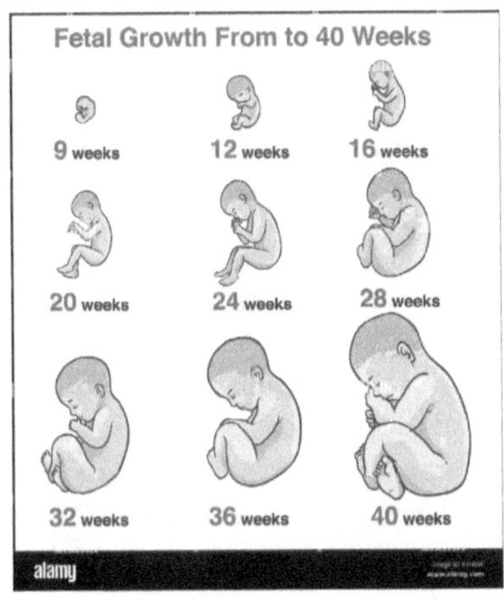

nced at the pamphlets she handed me. Options, I had options. One read Abortion, another
ption. My hands were shaking so bad I could barely see the information on the cover of each
phlet. She also handed me samples of prenatal vitamins, a list of local obstructions and a print out
e various stages of fetal development with what they assumed was mine circled. She explained
they based it off my questionnaire. circled was 12 weeks.

w" I said quietly,

ver missed my period.

recommended I make a doctor's appointment and ask that very question. The Grey-haired lady left
room so she could give me a few minutes alone to sit with my results. She told me I could leave
n I was ready. Before leaving the tiny office, she handed me a card with her phone number and ext.
t in case I had any further questions or concerns. I took all the papers, vitamins and business card,
fed them into my back pack and quickly left the Health Unit. Sitting there while I freaked out did not
m to make much sense. It would not change the fact that I was Pregnant.

lked around until I was certain school was over, trying to keep things as routine as possible, so that
n I returned home it would be at my normal time as If I had been in school all day. Hoping the
ool had not called home I reluctantly went home. Walking up the porch steps I could hear my mom
ming happily. That was not what I was expecting. I opened the door waiting for the anger and
ppointment, but there was none. My mom was happy. She smiled as I passed her. Gratefully, I
kly made my way to my room upstairs.

re were three rooms upstairs, one was my room which I shared with my sister Jean the other room
my brother's room then there was a small bathroom. As I passed my brother's room his door
ned, he was standing there not looking very happy. He informed me the school called, and he
ded to talk to me. I entered his room and plopped down on the end of his bed. I never made eye
tact. I just sat there staring at the floor, I waited for him to speak. He informed me the school called;
mom stepped out resulting in him picking up the phone. He took message but he never passed it
g and has been waiting to speak to me. Making sense of my mom's reaction, my brother demanded
now where I was, since I was not in school. Still avoiding eye contact I began to explain. He stood
ening quietly until I was finished speaking, he finally spoke. "You need to tell mom, and soon". I

agreed but not for a few months. I wanted to wait until after my 18th. birthday. I asked him to be wi
me for support when I did. He agreed.

Leaving my brother's room, I was exhausted. Entering my room, I placed my school bag by the end o
bed on the floor. Dropping into my bed, I began to drift off to sleep. I could hear the vibrating of my
phone as I laid there. Reaching for my bag I pulled out my phone. Crap!

I forgot to touch base with my friends to update them on how things went at the Health Uni
There were so many messages. I sent a quick text to each of them. "Test was Positive". Turning off n
cell without waiting for any replies, I plugged it into my wall charger and drifted off to sleep. Waking
three in the morning according to my alarm clock I noticed I had a blanket on and my shoes were ne
by my door. My mom must have come up. My tummy growled reminding me I did not have supper.
Rolling over I drifted off ignoring it. Dreaming great dreams of being carefree and young. The month
flew by

. My birthday came and went. We celebrated it in house with mom making n
favorite for supper and we had chocolate cake for dessert. Mom wanted to throw me a party, invitin
my friends from school and making my birthday a big deal. I requested to just celebrate with my fam
Disappointed she obliged.

With my birthday over it was time to tell my parents I was pregnant as I agreed to do. I waited until
there was a morning when my parents would be together at the same time in the same location. I
overheard my parents the night after we celebrated my 18th birthday making plans for the following
morning. I informed my brother and the plan to break the news to my parents about my pregnancy v
in motion. The following morning my brother offered to drive Jean and I to school, only Jean exited t
car when we arrived. I remained in the car so my brother could take me to speak with my parents. M
worked in a coffee shop down the street from our house. She worked part time hours to help pay the
bills.

Mom and dad had planned to go have something to eat and a coffee before mom started her shift th
day. As planned my brother pulled up to the school Jean hopped out before his car came to a comple
stop. Jean jogged over to her group of friends gathered near the front doors of the school She never
realized I stayed in the car. I watched her, so carefree. As my brother slowly drove off. We sat in sile
He made his way to the coffee shop where my mom worked. As we pulled into the parking lot my
parents were standing beside their van. My mom looked up locking eyes with me, scowling she cross
her arms.

brother directed me to get out and wait in the parking lot for him to park his car. Checking the
ket of my jeans to make sure I remembered to place the sheet with the stages of fetal development
my pocket I hesitated but did as he asked. As I stood there my mom began walking towards me. With
voice raised she insisted I explain why I was not in school. I stood there alone frozen like a deer
ght in head lights on a dark stretch of road. Where was my brother?

at was taking him so long?

re my only thoughts. Hearing the tone in my mom's voice and seeing me standing there looking
ified, my father made his way towards us.

t as my dad found his place beside my mom, my brother arrived to my location. I took a step back so I
s shielded by my brother's body, I reached into the front pocket of my jeans. Finding what I was
king for I leaned around my brother's body

handed my mom the sheet with the stages of fetal development to my mom. My mom took the
et, unfolding it she scanned it. After a few minutes she sighed and handed the sheet to my father.
father looked up from the sheet of paper after just a few minutes of looking at it and his words
cked me. "Are you hungry". He had noticed I did not eat much for breakfast that morning and
ered to buy me breakfast. Furious, my mom looked at him. His reason for his reaction was justified
h just five words. "At least she is not dead". I followed my dad inside the coffee shop and took my
t alone to eat while my parents talked at a separate table, my brother decided to wait in his car.

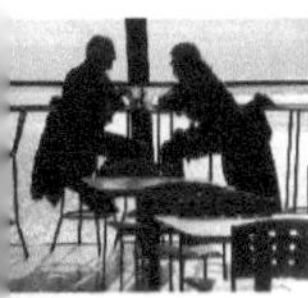

parents had decided that I would still attend school as long as i could. My pregnancy would be kept a
ret

ept from my friends knowing for now. During the first six months of my pregnancy my mom would
ite me notes to get out of school for Doctor's appointments or to get out of participating in physed
sses. She seemed to accept my pregnancy and even seemed excited she was going to be a grandma.
elt like almost Dailly I would come home from school to more and more baby supplies. My mom was
gain shopping.

d was working a lot; he seemed tired all the time. One night just around the six-month mark of my
egnancy I could hear my parents talking. My mom had noticed how tired my dad has been. She
gested he take a break even just a few days. Dad refused saying that a baby cost money and needed
t, that he could not. I felt so guilty but so grateful to have my parents helping me. At about six
nths pregnant it became more obvious and more difficult to hide the fact that I was pregnant. I could
ar the whispers as I passed groups of people standing in the hallways at school. I missed the days
en I was invisible. Ignoring them I made my way to my classes. One day we had a substitute for
tory Class, his name was Mr. Trow.

made it clear what his expectations were for his class before he started the class. One of his rules
s that we were not permitted to leave class for any reason unless ill or the office made a request for

us. Shortly after class began, I had to pee. Now with being pregnant one of its draw backs was the constant need to pee. My little one growing inside me liked to use my bladder as a dance matt to practice its moves and my baby was the star. Today was no different.

I put up my hand trying to patiently wait for the teacher to acknowledge it. Finally, he did. I made my request and as expected he denied it. Fidgeting in my seat, I attempted to hold my bladder. Realizing was losing that battle. I stood up by my desk. Loudly I announced I was pregnant not fat, and I really needed to pee. If the teacher refused, I was willing to walk up and relieve myself in his trash can besi his desk Infront of everyone. After announcing it i began to walk towards the trash can. In a Panick th teacher told me to just go. With my secret out of the bag it spread throughout the remainder of the like wild fire.

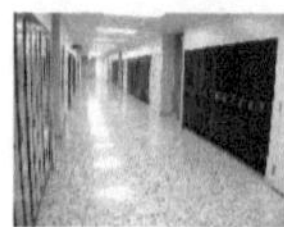

So much so later that night after we had just finished supper the home phone rang. My mom answer it, she nodded and hung it up. She informed me the principal would like to meet my parents and I the following morning. My dad mentioned he could not attend he had to work. It would be just my mom and me. Morning came fast. The principal was waiting for us when we arrived at the school. He direc me to a chair outside his

office then ushered my mom inside. I could not make out what they were saying but my mom did rai her voice several times. After some time, the office door opened and my mom walked past without saying a word. On instinct I followed her assuming I was supposed to and we left the school. On the v home she spoke not a word. I picked up on her wish for silence so I sat there saying nothing.

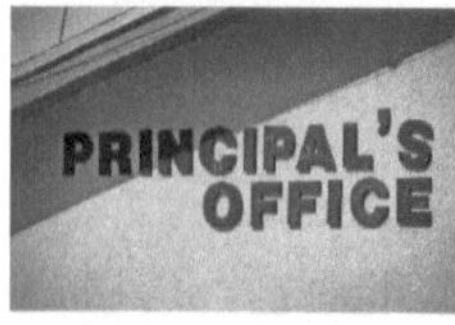

Once we were home my mom picked up the phone to call

my father. Over hearing their conversation I now understood why my mom had raised her voice in th principal's office. The principal's along with the Board of Education had decided that I would no longe attend school. I would finish my semester at home with a tutor coming to my parents' house paid for and provided by the school. They all felt my situation created a problem for the other students in the school. They were concerned that other girls would get pregnant too because I was. As if it was contagious. They did not want to take that risk and felt It best I no longer attend school. On top of tha was denied the ability to take graduation photos, with my class at school as it was felt to be a waste o school resources.

The school system assumed I would not complete school. That I would drop out to raise my baby like many before me did in my situation had done. They were supposed to be educators and felt I was a lo cause. I do not know if it was the hormones from pregnancy or if I was just angry at being labelled a statistic, but it lit a fire under me and for the next year i worked hard towards earning enough credits

duate high school. I spent the remainder of my semester working with the assigned tutor then signed
to receive book at home to complete additional work on my own. I did not have much contact with
friends. Not because we were not friends anymore but because word got out that I was pregnant,
their parents did not want them spending time with me anymore.

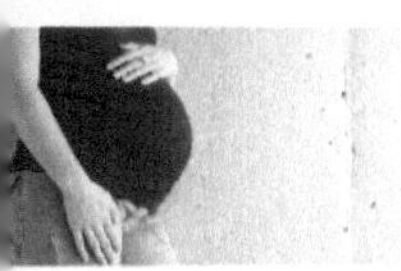

My time as a carefree teen was over. It was time to grow up and be responsible. As a teen you
as if you know all there is to know about being grown. Like you are ready to embark out on your
n. Truth was that we had no clue and were far from ready to be an adult with adult responsibilities.
mom gave me space to work, she was busy on her own end ensuring we had all we would need for
arrival of my baby, her grandbaby. After a lot of hard work and determination I succeeded. I had
ned enough credits to graduate high school. The principal was notified by the Board of Education
ulting in a telephone call to my parents.

mom answered the call that day. Calling me to the kitchen she informed me the principal phoned,
was impressed and wanted to let my parents and I know that I was able to attend graduation at the
ool if I would like. Shaking my head, NO, flat out refusing. To me my reasons were justified. The
ncipal and Board of Education had treated me poorly, judged me harshly and I did not want to have
thing to do with them. My mom as a result requested my diploma be mailed. Once it arrived, we
ebrated at home taking lots of pictures. I did it.

raduated Highschool.

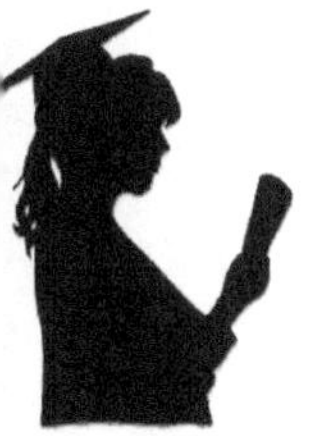

approximately eight months pregnant I left my Obstetricians' appointment feeling scared. Dr. Asher
ormed me mom and I that my baby was breached with the umbilical cord wrapped around its neck.
at that meant was my baby by a certain point in my pregnancy should be upside down with its feet
ar my ribs. This position prepares the baby a natural delivery.

If delivered natural under the current situation the umbilical cord would tighten during delivery cuttir

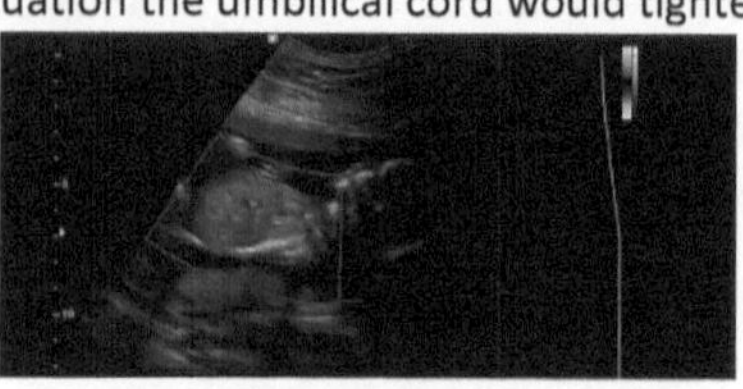

off my baby's oxygen resulting in death.

Delivering naturally was not safe. I would need a C-section. My mom must have noticed how terrified
was feeling as she places her hand on my arms assuring me all would be fine. She explained that she h
delivered my brother by c-section. She never explained why she had to deliver that way but knowing :
did and they were both ok made me feel better. She also made sure to remind me that stress was not
good for me or the baby I tried to calm down and think of something else. As we drove home, I thoug
of how much I missed my fog friends. It seemed so long ago since I spoke to them or saw them. I'll mu
adjust and learn to deal with things myself. My situation demands I try. I did not have anyone to confi
in accept my mom.

My sister Jean, now knowing I was pregnant, was cruel and always put me down. My brother was nev
home and my dad was always working. I had made the decision to rid Corey of any responsibility,
deciding it was best for my baby after falsely claiming that I had cheated on him. That resulted in him
cutting off all contact. Understandably It was difficult to break his heart like that but it was the right
decision for my baby's future. Mom did not agree or disagree with my decision to not have a father
involved she never spoke of her feelings about it at all. She just supported my decision and that was
that. I had trouble sleeping after the Doctor gave me the news about the possibility of my baby being
strangled by the umbilical cord. Not to mention the thought of having surgery.

The date was booked. December 14th. The only positive things about having a c-section were that I
knew exactly when my baby would be born, taking away the surprise portion of going into labor. That
also meant I would not be going into labor. I was going to be monitored to ensure I don't. I would not
shopping out with my mom one day and bam! Time.

In some ways that comforted me. Mom and I spent the next several weeks buying last minute baby
things. It was crazy how much someone so little needed. Finally, we were ready. At least I hoped we
were. Perfect timing as it was the day before surgery was to take place. Mom was packing up things fo
the hospital.

One of the items moms made sure to pack was an infant car seat. I questioned it because I did not hav
a license let alone drive. Why would I need an infant car seat. It made no sense. Can't I just bring a bu
and when the baby and I are discharged place it inside and make our way home. Mom informed me th

hospital rules state that to have my baby discharged into my care we must have an infant car seat to
 him home in.

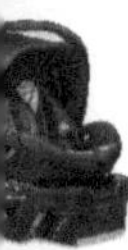

s are rules but I found that one odd, not everyone drives.

y in the morning On December 14th my mom woke me earlier than necessary. I was not due to be
ie hospital for another three hours. Unable to eat and only able to drink some water because I was
ng surgery, made me hangry. I was so miserable. It is not easy to tell my growing baby that I can't
won't be eating. I was being kicked like crazy and my tummy was talking. As I complained my mom
hed at me. It just frustrated me more. Being pregnant is hard on the body with your hormones on a
er coaster ride. Mom would often smile accepting my many moods. I never realized I was acting
erent or irrationally.

ne all my feelings were for good reasons. I woke up feeling sore my well, my everything was sore.
feet the rare time I could see them were always swollen my shoes or sandals did not fit. I wore
bers. My face was fat. I had two chins. I put on thirty pounds and it is considered a healthy weight
 for pregnancy and perfectly normal. I was hungry all the time and my boobs constantly hurt. The
 good part of it all was that I did not have to wear pads anymore. At least not the ones you stick to
r panties. Instead, I wore them in my bra. I never knew that breast pads were a thing.

    At a certain point in your pregnancy for some ladies or just after pregnancy boobs start to leak.
 It is a sign your body is preparing to breast feed. I did not read any of this in the pamphlet's the
lth Unit gave me that day I was told I was pregnant. I am pretty sure if they put some things like
ing thirty pounds and leaky boobs in the pamphlets it would be enough to deter young girls from
ing pregnant. I will admit that the weight gain was the most difficult to accept. I was a little vain. I
ss I did complain a lot.

parents had been great helping me through this and accepting me. My mom working hard to ensure
were ready and dad working until he was too tired to even have supper when he got home. I looked
t like my mom. Before I was pregnant of course. At least that is what I was often told when we were
 somewhere together. Mom stood about 5' 5" tall weighing 200 pounds with brown hair and brown
s. My dad was about 5' 10" inches tall with black salt and pepper hair, brown eyes and a chin that
embled Elvis Presley's. Well under his beard he did. Dad worked hard allowing mom to stay home to
e us kids. I hope I am as good as a mom as she is. "Time to go" yelled my mom. I was to be at the
pital in thirty minutes. Suddenly I snapped back into the her and now Panick took over. My insides
e vibrating. My dad helped me put on my slippers. It was difficult, I was so round reaching my feet
 a chore and I could not get them to just slip on. Damn things.

lowed my parents out to their van. It was packed and ready ahead of time. My legs were so unsteady
 shaking so badly I was surprised they held me up. It was December and winter time. There was a
t dusting of snow on the ground lightly covering but not hiding my parents' van. It was not cold
ept the odd gust of wind. Man, that wind was cold. Climbing into the back seat I grabbed a nearby
nket my mom kept in the van and huddled under it.

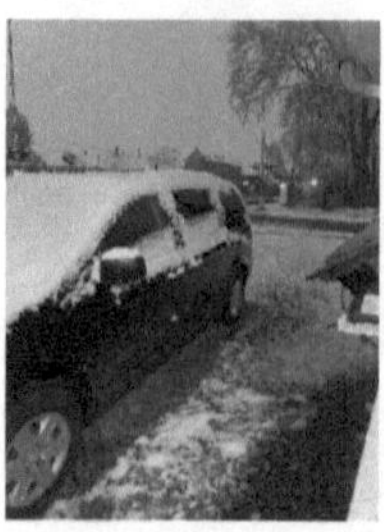

Mom played the radio low and talked about random things like spring flowers she wanted to plant ir
garden after the Winter had passed. Mom loved to be out in the yard working away in the garden wh
spring hit. She took pride in her home and worked to keep it nice. Our house was white two floors w
large fenced in yard. It had four bedrooms but one was used for my dad's office. He ran a drywall
business from our house and it was mandatory he have a home office. Something to do with taxes o
the government. The house sat nestled next to the train tracks so that whenever the train passed th
house should shake a little. Living there you got used to it to the point where you never noticed it. If
friends slept over, they would complain about the train shaking the house and being noisy.

As we drove to the hospital my mom kept glancing at me in her rearview mirror. I smiled pretending
nod along to the music. In truth I was not really listening to it. Inside I was a ball of nerves. On arrival
mom parked in the hospital parking lot paying for a day. She obviously expected to be there for a lor
time. Dad unpacked the van trailing behind mom and I. We made our way to the first elevators on ot
right as we entered the front doors of the hospital. Mom had a sheet that directed her where to go. I
have no idea where that sheet came from or when she was given it. Entering the elevator, she presse
the button for the third floor and the elevator creaked and groan like the weight inside was too muck
for it.

Slowing to a stop the elevator moaned. The metal doors complained as they opened. I wondered how
safe it was for people to be taking anywhere in the hospital, let alone someone pregnant. Infront of
was an L shaped desk. Several women in hospital scrubs were seated at various computer monitor's
typing away. None of them looked up to acknowledge our arrival. My mom

cleared her throat as she approached the desk to try and get someone's attention. After a few minut
of waiting mom grew a little impatient. As a result, she just blurted out the reason we were standing
there to anyone that may be listening. She placed her registration papers on the desk she had brougł
from home tapping her fingers beside them. Growing impatient she proceeded to speak to whomeve
may be listening and informed them why were there A young woman maybe in her early twenties str
up smiling as she walked towards my mom. She stopped on her way to grab what appeared to be a
digital pad of some sort.

She had a patch on the left sleeve of her scrub top with the name of a college on it and the word stur
printed on it. She asked my mom questions and typed in some information. Satisfied, she instructed
to follow her. Taking us down a long hallway with many doors. I could hear babies crying from inside
several. All accept one. On the outside of that door was a purple butterfly. Mom saw me looking at it
and leaning over she explained what it meant. She told me that the butterfly let hospital staff know t
the mom inside had an angel baby. Born but not living or that passed away shortly after birth.

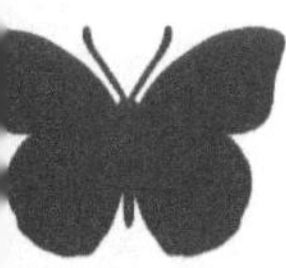

w sad. Carry your baby filled with worry and excitement. Planning for your new future. Pick a name, up a nursery and fill your home with all the things your new bundle could possibly need. But will er use. You come home empty. My heart broke for her. A mom in mourning. I could not imagine ng through all that I have to end up with nothing afterwards. My mom seeing the look on my face d the tears in my eyes reassure me I had nothing to worry about. The Doctor was confident rything would be fine. I still could not help but worry. My mom worried all the time. I guess it is part being a mom. Our nurse stopped in front of an open door it was just a few doors down from the door t had the butterfly on it. She handed me a hospital gown she had taken off a cart in the hallway. She owed with instructions to put the gown on then wait in the room. A porter would be down to get me rtly to take me to the operating room.

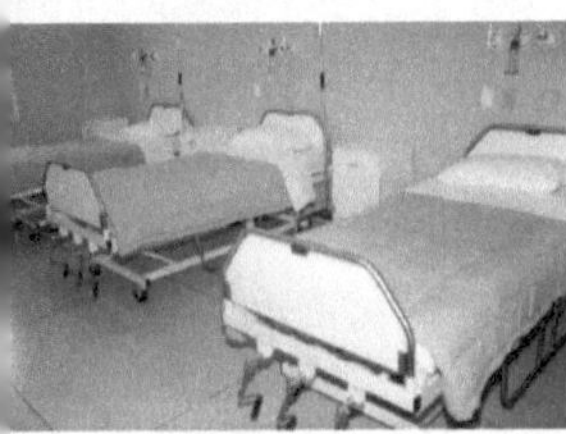

orter is someone whose main job is to pick up patients from their rooms and ensure they get to the ation throughout the hospital for tests or to be taken to surgery. My dad left the room with my mom go get a coffee to give me privacy to change. I drew the curtain that hung from the ceiling shielding bed from the other four that were empty in my room and put on the gown. My room was called a rd room. They were rooms shared with four to six other people. They were for people that did not ve private insurance or that did not pay for a private room. Private rooms were expensive and dad s an independent contractor so we had no health insurance accept the insurance provided by our vernment for being a citizen. I did not mind sharing a room. I did at home anyway.

onder once home how the room situation will be worked out. Will Jean and I continue to share a m and my baby will join us or will mom and dad arrange something else?

n not sure how that will work out. I am sure my mom has a plan. Mom and dad were so busy packing van that morning and making sure they had everything ready neither took time to have a coffee or . So, while I got ready, they took the opportunity to pick up a coffee. It was like liquid gold to my rents. A necessary part of starting each day. I did not personally like the taste but I wondered if as an ult I would. Like it was a taste I would not appreciate until I was an adult. Shortly after I was gowned d seated on the hospital bed in my room the hospital assigned me. My parents were back. Trailing em was short stocky guy with a name tag I could not make out. He announced he was my porter igned to take me to surgery.

He instructed me to lay on the bed I was already seated on. He needed to wheel me to another floor. asked to walk but due to hospital rules I was not allowed. The reason is if I was to fall walking and inj myself or my unborn child, I could sue the hospital for a lot of money. To avoid that I was to remain i the bed or be placed in a wheel chair when being portered to various locations in the hospital.

 Hugging my parents, I laid back and off we went. Out the door left down the hallway towards the elevator doors. As he wheeled me down the hall, I felt the remanent of my childhood fade away. It w bitter sweet. I quietly said goodbye to my childhood. Embracing this new chapter in my life I took a d breath and attempted to clear my mind.

The attempt to clear my mind was not easy. Instead, I let it wander. I thought of how strange it was t my pregnancy had somehow made my mom and I closer. It was something we never had before. On different level. The elevator took us down to the basement. When the doors opened the words, surg were in clearly written on a sign. The porter parked my bed in in the hallway just past the elevators across from an open door. He explained that they were ensuring my room was ready for surgery. Onc the doors were closed it would be a sterilized field and they are not supposed to open them again un surgery was complete. He informed me that someone will be with me shortly and congratulated me before he walked away.

After several long minutes a nurse came out of the room across from me. She stopped at my bed a asked If I had been prepped for surgery yet. I told her what took place up to this point and she nodde Crouching down she unlocked the wheels of the bed I was on and wheeled me a few doors down. Opening the door, she pushed my bed inside. I was in a small room. It contained a chair, a sink, a counter with cotton swabs, white wash cloths and a large floor light. She took a seat explaining she h to shave the area where the Doctor's were going to cut. It had to be clean and free of any body hair. Then she directed me as to where she would shave.

She acted like it was work as usual. I found it awkwardly uncomfortable. The nurse needed to shave o the top Portion of my Pubic hair. I laid there for the first time in months having difficulty getting my mind to wander. So, I would not concentrate on what was taking place at that moment. With the task done I was wheeled back into the hallway where I waited. Pregnancy was a lot of waiting and did not allow very much privacy or dignity.

As I laid there waiting on my bed in the hallway My Porter returned. He passed me and entered my would-be surgery room. He was holding a digital pad when he entered and empty handed when he exited. He smiled and was gone. Man, he was quick. I guess he would have to be. The hospital was lar and from what I gathered on arrival very busy.

I could hear a clunking noise followed by footsteps out of view approaching me. Appearing ahead was nurse with navy blue scrubs on. She was pushing a cart. As she got closer, I saw the cart's contents. It looked to be medieval torture devices gleaming the hallway lights. Worse yet she pushed that cart of torture into my operating room If I could get off this bed and run I would. But I have not done much running in months. The torture devices reminded me of ones I have seen on some old horror movies. After a few minutes the lady in navy blue scrubs reappeared and walked towards me.

She smiled, bent over, unlocked the wheels of my bed and maneuvered my bed into the
erating room across the hall. Inside the room were large lights, some were mounted to the ceiling,
ers on metal arms mounted to the walls. The cart of torture was parked beside a narrow shiny metal
d. There is no way that bed is meant for me. Just at first glance my size compared to the size of that
d did not seem like a realistic fit. The room reminded of those emergency 911 shows. The ones that
 fictional. I was impressed with how realistic they managed to get their operating rooms. The only
ng missing was all the drama. It was eerily quiet.

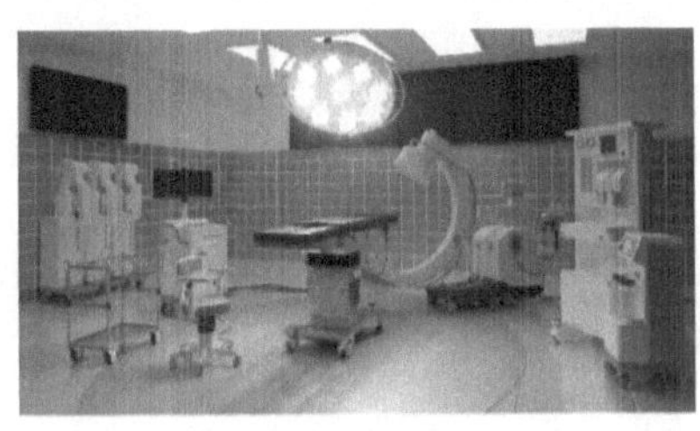

nust have said some of what I was thinking out loud as I heard Dr. Asher from somewhere in the room
rt to laugh. It was hard to tell which person standing in the room was him. Everyone had a hospital
ub cap and mask on. just a bunch of eyes gathered in the room. But I recognized the sound of his
gh. One of the people with eyes in the room asked me to slide onto the shiny metal tiny bed. I replied
h an exaggerated OK. Reluctantly giving up my comfy wide long bed for the shiny thin one. i was sure
 idea of this bed was not well thought out when the room was designed. I moved with zero grace or
gance. After laying down I felt like I was hanging off the bed in every direction. I was then strapped
wn to the bed with my arms at my sides. comfort was not at all possible. Good news. I fit...

Asher's voice rang out like the captain of a ship. He commanded the room in full control. A person
ned into my view appearing upside down. The upside-down person with the eyes placed a rubber
sk I recognized is used for oxygen over my face and asked me to count backwards starting at ten. The
t number I remember saying was I think six, then everything went black.

en I woke up my mouth was dry. It felt like I swallowed a bunch of cotton balls. Or at least how I
agined my mouth would feel had I swallowed some. My body was kind of numb and hurt just a little
the same time. I could hear a fan ruffling papers each time it passed them. There was a beeping noise
 some monitors to my left. I could not see anyone but I am sure someone had to be nearby. I
empted to speak but all I could manage was a groan. My mind was alert but my body was not in tune
h it. Shortly after I groaned, I could hear footsteps. A tall thin woman with a pointed nose and thin
s appeared at my bedside. As if she teleported in. I could still hear footsteps so obviously they were
t hers.

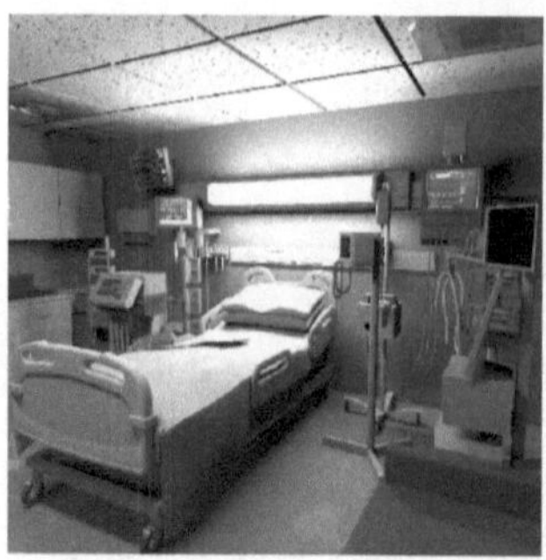

She had a drink in hand. A plastic cup with a straw in it. I have no idea what I drank but it was so good. Sweet. She checked my blood pressure, listened to my heart then left the room. When she returned Asher was with her. He did the same things she had done before leaving and during the checkup he informed me that my surgery went well. I had been asleep for some time and he was beginning to worry. Convinced I was fine. He followed with "You have a son; He is doing very well". I thanked him before he left my bedside. The nurse explained she was going to give me a little longer for the sedation from surgery to wear off then she would have my porter wheel me to my room. I nodded and closed eyes for a little longer. I was woken up by my porter unlocking the wheels of my bed. Looking around realized I was in my big wide long comfy bed again. Gratefully I just laid there in silence as he wheeled me out of the room, I could only assume was recovery.

Recovery is where patients go after procedures to rest and wait sedation to wear off. They are monitored before being cleared to go home or to their hospital room that was assigned to them. I felt my bed hit something. Opening my eyes, I realized it was the door to my room. It was partly closed and he was using my bed to push it open while pushing my bed inside. As we entered, I saw my mom seated in a chair on her cell phone stuffing her face with one my favorite donuts holding a coffee in her hand. She smiled, hung up her cell phone emptying her hands she stood up.

Once my porter locked my wheels after putting my bed in its proper location he was off again. A nurse entered the room just as he was leaving. My mom said something I could not hear to her and she left again. Shortly after she returned pushing a cart with a plastic tub attached to the top. Inside the tub was blue baby blankets and a tiny head with a hat on it peeking out from under the blankets. My heart was racing. My mom was standing and smiling. Her eyse twinkling. She looked excited, so happy. She announced how beautiful he was. He was healthy and doing so good. She leaned down hugged me, being careful not to squeeze. I did just have abdominal surgery and even though the pain was minor right now it was a major surgery. The only reason the pain was minor was the fact I was on a lot of pain medication.

My son, a boy. I had never really thought of what I wanted. A boy or a girl. I never really thought about it. i did pick out a name for each. Mind you, the name I had picked for a boy if I had one was changed. My dad being religious had believed that God spoke to him after a near collision with a transport truck that would have surely taken his life. God told him I was going to have a boy and even named him. At first, I argued and fought the name. But after some time, I decided to go with it. Boy or girl did not matter just a healthy living baby was all I wanted.

I was a mom!

ole to hold him right away, I grew irritable. I needed a nurse to either take away or situate some of wires and tubes that were still attached to me. One was to monitor my heart rate there was a blood sure cuff that was still inflating on my right upper arm. I had an IV and my tubes were tangled in the of my bed. The nurse explained that all but my iv should have been removed in recovery and logized. She removed and untangled things. Freeing me up a little more. Afterwards I asked my mom he nurse if I could hold my son. My mom went to lift him and the nurse stopped her. Hospital Policy es the nurse must lift him out the bassinet she called the plastic tub he was in if a nurse was present he room at the time. Another odd rule. My mom, disappointed stepped back dropping her arms to sides. Allowing room for the nurse to reach in and pick up my little miracle. As she placed him into arms, she repositioned my arms so I could hold him. After showing me how she called my mom over he bed in case I needed any assistance. I did not even see the nurse leave my room. As I held Him fell erfectly in love with him. I never felt love like I did in that moment ever before.

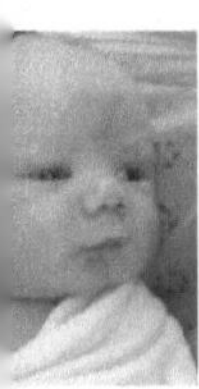

t so lucky. Like I just received the greatest gift.

n December 14th. On a winter day with a light dusting of snow on the ground was my perfect azing tiny human. As I sat up in my hospital bed holding him in my arms while staring down at him, I ized that this very moment is why I existed. It was to bring this little guy into this world. In my arms I d the future. Part of me lives in him. What an amazing journey.

m Birth to Rebirth. Truth is my journey has just begun.